Bird Flu Mysteries

A Comprehensive Guide to Understanding, Mitigating, And Safeguarding Against Avian Influenza

Judith Bell

Table of Contents

Introduction

Bringing to Light the Danger: An Overview of the Bird Flu

An infectious viral infection that mostly affects birds, including both farmed poultry and wild birds, is referred to as avian influenza, which is also widely referred to as bird flu. In addition to being a member of the influenza A virus family, the virus is further subdivided into a number of different subtypes depending on the combination of surface proteins, hemagglutinin (H), and neuraminidase (N). Particularly, the H5N1 and H7N9 subtypes have garnered a lot of attention because to the fact that they are linked to severe sickness in birds and can occasionally be transmitted to humans.

Transmission

- Bird-to-Bird: The most common way that avian influenza is transmitted from bird to bird is through direct contact with infected birds, as well as through their saliva, nasal secretions, and bodily waste.

- Zoonotic Potential: Certain strains of avian influenza have the potential to infect people, typically through intimate contact with infected birds or the settings in which they live.

Variants and Strains

There are many different strains and subtypes of avian influenza, with H5N1 and H7N9 being of particular concern due to the impact they have on the health of both birds and humans.

Effects on Birds

Avian influenza can cause serious sickness in domestic chickens, which can result in high death rates and economic losses for the poultry industry. Avian influenza can also cause severe illness in wild birds. It is possible for wild birds, particularly ducks, to carry and spread the virus although they do not exhibit any symptoms.

Although the majority of strains of avian influenza do not infect humans, certain subtypes of the virus, when transmitted to humans, can cause serious respiratory illness and, in some instances, even death.

Concerns Regarding the Pandemic

The propensity of avian influenza viruses to undergo genetic reassortment raises worries about the formation of novel strains that have the potential for effective human-to-human transmission, which might lead to a pandemic that affects the entire world.

Prevention and Control

Vaccination, stringent biosecurity measures, and the culling of sick birds are some of the strategies that can be utilized to control avian influenza in poultry.

Monitoring and surveillance of wild bird populations are important components of early detection and containment efforts.

Avian influenza is a global concern because of the impact it has on the health of both humans and animals, the economic repercussions it has, and the possibility that it could be transmitted internationally. International collaboration is absolutely necessary for the purposes of surveillance, the exchange of information, and the coordination of responses to outbreaks.

When it comes to avoiding and managing outbreaks, minimizing economic losses, and protecting public health, having a solid understanding of the dynamics of avian influenza is absolutely necessary.

Historical Perspectives: Past Outbreaks and Lessons Learned

The historical context of avian influenza is a convoluted story that is intricately intertwined with the interaction that exists between people and domesticated birds, notably poultry. Over the course of several decades, the history of avian influenza unfolds, with significant events and discoveries influencing our comprehension of this viral danger from the beginning.

Beginnings and Initial Appearances

When scientists and veterinarians first started seeing unexplained outbreaks of respiratory disorders in domestic poultry at the beginning of the 20th century, this is when the beginnings of avian influenza can be traced back to. On the other hand, until more sophisticated diagnostic methods became available, the true nature of these outbreaks remained a mystery.

First Case Identified: In 1959, Scotland was the location where the first case of avian influenza was discovered and identified. The virus was isolated from a flock of turkeys, which was a critical milestone in the process of establishing the unique characteristics of avian influenza as a viral infection in birds.

The puzzle of avian influenza was gradually stitched together by scholars throughout the middle of the 20th century. This was the third step in the evolution of understanding. The researchers became aware that the virus could infect a wide variety of bird species, including chickens, ducks, and turkeys, and they were able to identify multiple strains of the virus, each of which possessed its own distinct properties.

The H5N1 outbreak that occurred in Hong Kong in 1997 is considered to be one of the most significant events in the history of avian influenza. It was discovered that the H5N1 strain of the virus had spread from birds to humans, which led to a number of instances of the virus in humans and a significant mortality rate. The zoonotic potential of avian influenza was brought to the attention of people all around the world as a result of this tragedy.

The spread of avian influenza occurred over the latter part of the 20th century and the early 21st century. Enhanced international commerce and travel played a significant role in facilitating the transmission of the virus across continents. There was an increase in the number of outbreaks that occurred in chicken farms and wild bird populations, which presented difficulties in terms of containment and control.

The H1N1 influenza pandemic that occurred in 2009 brought to light the ability of influenza viruses to undergo reassortment and hop between different species. The dynamic nature of avian influenza viruses and their potential to pose severe public health concerns were brought to light by this incident.

Over the past few years, our understanding of avian influenza has been enhanced by continuous surveillance, research, and developments in molecular biology. By conducting genomic investigations, scientists are able to monitor the evolution of various strains, forecast the occurrence of possible pandemics, and devise control measures that are specifically targeted.

It is vital to gain an understanding of the historical context of avian influenza in order to gain useful insights into the problems that are faced by this viral threat. From its humble beginnings as a mysterious poultry disease to its global influence on public health, avian influenza continues to be a dynamic and developing challenge that requires continual scientific investigation and international collaboration. This is because both of these factors are necessary for addressing the issue.

There was an increase in awareness of the zoonotic potential of avian influenza, which led to an increase in surveillance at the interface between humans and animals.

As a result of the interconnected nature of the modern world, global collaboration has become an essential component in the process of monitoring, reporting, and responding to outbreaks. The lessons learned from previous epidemics highlighted the significance of pandemic readiness, which in turn prompted multinational efforts to produce vaccinations and antiviral treatments.

For the purpose of formulating successful strategies for future preventive, control, and response activities, it is of the utmost importance to have a thorough understanding of the historical perspectives of avian influenza outbreaks. The progression of our knowledge, beginning with the earliest observations and continuing up to the present day, is a reflection of the dynamic nature of this viral menace as well as the continual commitment to ensuring the safety of world health.

The Science Behind Bird Flu.

Avian Influenza Virus: Structure and Function

It is vital to have a solid understanding of the structure and function of the avian influenza virus in order to have a complete comprehension of its behavior, transmission, and the possible impact it can have on human populations as well as bird populations in some instances.

Structure of the Virus

1. Envelope and Surface Proteins: - The avian influenza virus is enveloped, and it has a lipid bilayer that is derived from the membrane of the host cell. - Surface proteins are included in the envelope. Hemagglutinin (referred to as H) and neuraminidase (referred to as N) are two essential surface proteins that play important roles in the process of viral entry and departure.

2. The Hemagglutinin (H) Protein: The H protein is responsible for facilitating the attachment of the virus to the cells of the host.

Within the context of determining the host range of the virus and its capacity to infect a variety of species, it is an extremely important factor.

3. Neuraminidase (N) Protein: The N protein plays a role in the release of new virions from cells that have been infected with another virus. It prevents freshly generated virus particles from aggregating, which is a factor that contributes to the virus's progression.

4. Genetic Material (RNA): Single-stranded RNA is the form in which the genetic information of the avian influenza virus is carried. RNA is the material that is responsible for carrying genetic information. All of the critical proteins that are required for the virus to replicate and continue to exist are encoded in the viral genome.

Function of the Virus

1. Infection of Host Cells: The first step in the life cycle of a virus is the attachment of the H protein to sialic acid receptors that are located on the surface of

host cells. - It is subsequently through the process of endocytosis that the virus is able to enter the cell. This procedure is made possible by the fusion activity of the H protein.

2. Replication and Transcription: Once the virus has entered the host cell, the viral RNA is released and acts as a template for the process of replication and transcription. Both fresh viral RNA copies and viral proteins are produced throughout the process of viral synthesis.

3. Assembly and Budding: Newly synthesized viral components are delivered to the cell surface, where they assemble into new virions. Budding occurs when the viral components interact with the cell surface. During the process of budding, the N protein plays a role in facilitating the release of these virions from the host cell.

4. Evasion of the Host Immune System: The avian influenza virus possesses mechanisms that allow it to avoid being attacked by the immune system of the host. Certain antigenic variations, in particular those found in the H and N proteins, make it possible for the

virus to avoid being recognized by the immune system of the host.

Possible Zoonotic Effects

1. Adaptation and Zoonosis: The capacity of avian influenza viruses to adapt to a variety of host species is a significant component in determining the zoonotic potential of these viruses. There are certain strains of influenza that have demonstrated the ability to spread from birds to people, which can result in zoonotic illnesses. These strains include H5N1 and H7N9.

2. Reassortment: Avian influenza viruses are capable of undergoing genetic reassortment, which involves the exchange of genetic material with different influenza viruses. - This process has the potential to result in the creation of novel strains that have the capability of transmitting the disease from person to human in an effective manner.

To develop tactics for detection, prevention, and control of the avian influenza virus, both in bird populations and to limit the risks of zoonotic transmission to people, it is necessary to have a foundational understanding of the intricate interplay that exists between the structure and function of the virus.

Transmission Dynamics: How Bird Flu Spreads

Additionally, the dynamics of transmission of bird flu, also known as avian influenza, play a significant part in the propagation of the virus across avian populations and, in certain instances, in the transfer of the virus to human beings. The implementation of effective control measures and the reduction of the impact of outbreaks are both dependent on having a solid understanding of these dynamics on hand.

Avian-to-avian transmission

1. Direct touch: The most common way for the avian influenza virus to move from bird to bird is by humans coming into direct touch with sick birds. This can take place in a variety of contexts, such as inside flocks,

around water sources, or during gatherings of migrating birds from different locations.

2. Respiratory Secretions: The virus is found in respiratory secretions, such as nasal discharge and saliva, making close contact a crucial method of transmission. Birds that are infected excrete the virus through their respiratory droplets, which can then infect other birds that are susceptible to the infection.

3. The Fecal-Oral Route: The virus is also shed in feces, which contributes to the fecal-oral route of transmission. The virus can also be transmitted through the mouth. In the event that uninfected birds come into contact with infected excreta, interaction with contaminated feed, water, or surfaces can facilitate the transmission of the disease.

Migration of Wild Birds

The wild bird reservoir is a natural reservoir for avian influenza viruses, particularly waterfowl. Wild birds, in particular, are a reservoir for the virus. While migrating, wild birds that are infected with the virus have the potential to spread it to other geographical areas.

The virus is able to reside in water and on surfaces, both of which contribute to its ability to remain in the environment.

When exposed to polluted water sources or surfaces, birds that are not infected with the virus have the potential to get it.

Human-to-Avian Transmission

It has been established that certain strains of avian influenza, such as H5N1 and H7N9, have the capability to infect humans. This is referred to as the zoonotic potential. Direct contact with diseased birds or the surroundings in which they live can result in the spread of the disease from humans to birds.

Variables That Have an Effect on Transmission

Host Range and Susceptibility: The host range of avian influenza is controlled by the specific strain of the virus as well as the susceptibility of different types of birds.

It is possible for various strains to display varying degrees of pathogenicity by infecting different kinds of birds.

Environmental Factors: The parameters of the environment, such as temperature and humidity, can have an effect on the virus's ability to survive in the environment.

Conditions that are cold and rainy may be favorable for the virus to continue to exist.

Difficulties in Keeping Control

There is a possibility that the *international movement of chickens and poultry products* can contribute to the spread of avian influenza across international borders. This is a consequence of globalization and trade. In order to effectively adopt and enforce control measures, global trade presents a number of obstacles.

Asymptomatic Carriers: It is possible for certain birds to carry and shed the virus without producing any clinical indications, which makes it more difficult to detect and isolate those who are infected with the virus.

Control Measures

Biosecurity Practices: It is essential to implement stringent biosecurity measures in poultry farms in order to prevent and control the transfer of diseases. Controlling access, disinfecting, and conducting surveillance are all included in the measures.

Vaccination: Vaccinating chickens against particular strains of avian influenza is a preventative measure that can lessen the severity of the effects of outbreaks.

For the purpose of devising targeted and successful techniques to reduce the spread of the virus among avian populations and, if applicable, to prevent its transmission to humans, it is essential to have a comprehensive understanding of the complex dynamics of avian influenza transmission. In order to address the challenges that are posed by this viral threat, this multidimensional approach comprises a combination of biosecurity measures, surveillance, and international collaboration.

Strains and Variants: Navigating the Diversity of Avian Influenza.

Avian influenza, often known as bird flu, features a wide variety of strains and variations that are found within the influenza A virus family. This diversity is a reflection of the diversity of avian influenza. In order to comprehend the various properties of different strains, their influence on avian and human populations, and the development of effective measures for detection, prevention, and control, it is essential to be able to navigate this complexity.

Hierarchical Organization

The surface proteins hemagglutinin (H) and neuraminidase (N) are used to categorize the various types of influenza viruses that are found in birds.

Several different subtypes of H and N are present, which leads to a wide variety of combinations (for example, H5N1 and H7N9).

Strains are frequently named according to the geographical place where they were discovered, the species that those strains affected, and the chronological sequence in which they were identified.

The Most Important Strains of Avian Influenza

- *H5N1:* H5N1, one of the most well-known strains, drew attention all over the world due to the fact that it is highly pathogenic in birds and has the ability to infect people. The H5N1 virus has been responsible for catastrophic epidemics in poultry as well as sporadic occurrences in humans having significant fatality rates.
- *H7N9:* Another significant strain, H7N9, has shown zoonotic potential with sporadic human infections. - H7N9 has been linked to sporadic human infections. The fact that human cases frequently require exposure to infected poultry raises concerns about the potential for the disease to become a pandemic.

Variant characteristics include the following:

Pathogenicity: The pathogenicity of different strains of avian influenza can range from low to high, depending on the influenza strain

High-pathogenic strains have the potential to cause severe sickness, rapid spread, and huge economic losses via the chicken industry.

Zoonotic Potential: Certain strains have a higher zoonotic potential, which means that they have the ability to infect people. One of the most common ways that zoonotic transmission occurs is through intimate contact with diseased birds or habitats that are contaminated.

The Diversity of Genetics

Genetic reassortment: Avian influenza viruses are capable of undergoing *genetic reassortment*, which is a process in which various strains of the virus exchange genetic material with one another. The process of reassortment can result in the growth of novel strains that exhibit traits that are difficult to anticipate.

Evolutionary Changes: The genetic diversity of avian influenza is a factor that contributes to its capacity to adapt and evolve. Understanding the dynamic nature of the virus requires careful monitoring of the changes that occur in its genetic makeup.

Influence on the Populations of Avian Species

High-pathogenic avian influenza strains have the potential to create disastrous epidemics in poultry farms, which can lead to the culling of animals, limitations on trade, and economic losses.

Also, the wide variety of strains of avian influenza has ecological repercussions, as it has an effect on wild bird populations and the functioning of avian ecosystems.

Methods for Early Detection and Continuous Monitoring

Surveillance Programs: To monitor the prevalence and evolution of avian influenza strains in both domestic and wild bird populations, it is vital to have surveillance programs that are conducted on a regular basis.

Genomic Studies: Genomic studies allow researchers to examine the genetic composition of various strains, which enables them to get insights about the origins, evolution, and potential dangers of these strains.

To successfully navigate the wide variety of strains and types of avian influenza, which is a persistent problem, demands constant awareness, international cooperation, and a methodology that incorporates multiple disciplines. Scientists and health officials are able to better anticipate and respond to the ever-changing nature of this viral danger if they have a thorough understanding of the different characteristics of each strain.

The Impact on Avian Populations.

Avian Ecology: How Bird Flu Affects Wild Bird Species

The impact of avian influenza on wild bird species is the result of a complex interaction between the virus, the ecology of birds, and broader environmental conditions. A comprehensive understanding of the ways in which bird flu affects wild birds is essential for the conservation of wildlife, the maintenance of ecological balance, and the evaluation of the possible risk of transmission to domestic poultry and, in some instances, to humans.

Natural Reservoirs and Transmission.

Wild Bird Reservoir: Wild birds, particularly waterfowl like ducks and geese, act as natural reservoirs for avian influenza viruses. Wild birds are capable of transmitting the virus to humans. It is common for these birds to carry the virus without exhibiting any clinical symptoms, which contributes to the virus's ability to persist in the environment.

Migration Patterns: The migratory behavior of a great number of wild bird species makes it easier for the avian influenza virus to spread across wide geographical areas. During the courses of their seasonal migrations, infected birds have the potential to spread the virus to other places.

Clinical Signs and the Severity of the Disease.

Subclinical illnesses: A significant number of wild birds that have been infected with avian influenza display subclinical illnesses, which means that they do not exhibit any obvious signs of sickness. Because of this, it is difficult to detect and monitor the existence of the virus in populations of wild birds.

Severe Outcomes: Although wild birds can carry the virus without causing any obvious harm, specific strains of the virus have the potential to cause severe sickness and death in certain species, particularly waterfowl.

The Evolution of Ecosystems.

Population Dynamics: Outbreaks of avian influenza have the potential to alter the population dynamics of wild bird species. Localized decreases may occur as a consequence of severe outbreaks, which can have an impact on the abundance and distribution of species that are impacted.

Behavioral abnormalities: Birds that have been infected with the disease may display behavioral abnormalities, such as decreased eating or altered migration habits. Ecological relationships and the dynamics of communities may be affected as a result of these changes.

Transmission to Domestic Poultry

The Interaction with Domesticated Birds: Wild birds have the potential to act as a conduit for the transmission of avian influenza between natural reservoirs and farmed poultry. The close proximity of poultry farms to the habitats of wild birds creates the potential for the spread of diseases to domesticated birds.

The transmission of avian influenza from wild birds to domestic poultry can have serious repercussions for the economy, including the imposition of trade restrictions, the slaughter of domestic poultry, and economic losses.

Monitoring and Surveillance of the Situation.

Wildlife Surveillance Programs: It is absolutely necessary to have surveillance programs in place in order to monitor the population of wild birds for the presence of avian influenza. Both sampling and testing are helpful in determining whether or not the virus is present and whether or not it has the ability to spread to other species.

Conservation Obstacles and Challenges

Concerns Regarding Conservation: Outbreaks of avian influenza present difficulties for wildlife conservation efforts, particularly for species that are already confronted with problems such as the loss of habitat and climate change.

Striking a Balance Between Conservation and Disease Control: It is a difficult undertaking to find a balance between the conservation of wildlife and the measures used to control diseases. The elimination of sick birds in order to contain outbreaks may be incompatible with conservation objectives.

Research and the Approach of One Health Method.

The purpose of the ongoing research that is being conducted is to gain a more in-depth understanding of the ecology of avian influenza in wild birds. This includes the factors that influence transmission as well as the genetic diversity of the virus.

The One Health approach, which considers the interconnection of human, animal, and environmental health, is vital for addressing the complex dynamics of avian influenza in the wild.

It is necessary to take a holistic approach that takes into consideration ecological, behavioral, and epidemiological elements in order to gain an understanding of how bird flu affects wild bird species. Maintaining a balance between the conservation of wildlife and the control of disease is critical for the health of ecosystems and the well-being of both wild and domesticated bird populations. This is especially important as attempts to reduce the impact of avian influenza continue.

Poultry Industry Challenges: Economic Implications of Outbreaks

The poultry business faces significant economic hurdles at the hands of avian influenza epidemics, which have an impact on production, trade, and the stability of the market respectively. In order for stakeholders, politicians, and industry participants to successfully traverse the intricacies of managing and minimizing the impact of these outbreaks, it is essential for them to have a solid understanding of the economic ramifications.

Mortality and the Practice of Culling

Avian influenza, particularly the highly virulent strains, has the potential to cause considerable fatality rates among chicken flocks that are afflicted with the disease. In order to prevent the spread of the virus, control techniques frequently require preemptive culling, which results in the loss of entire flocks of animals.

Unexpected Disruptions to Production

The poultry supply chain is disrupted as a result of culling and mobility limitations, which in turn will have an effect on the production and distribution of chicken products.

We have a decreased capacity for production: On farms that have flocks that are affected, there is a possibility that production capacity may be lowered, which would result in a temporary decrease in overall output.

Trade restrictions

Trade restrictions are imposed on poultry products originating from impacted regions when outbreaks occur, which has an effect on worldwide exports. There are also obstacles that poultry producers must overcome in order to recover access to markets, which hinders their capacity to take part in international trade.

Problems with the Economy

Poultry farmers have direct financial losses as a result of decreased productivity, increased mortality, and the expense of applying biosecurity measures. There are also charges that are associated with cleaning and disinfection, testing, and the implementation of biosecurity policies that are considered indirect costs.

Confidence of the Consumer

Concerns Raised by Customers: It is possible that outbreaks will cause consumers to lose confidence in chicken products, even in places that are not immediately affected by the outbreak. It is possible that consumers will move their preferences toward alternate sources of protein, which will have an effect on the demand for the long-term market.

Industry-wide Impact

Producers of various sizes, both large and small: There are obstacles that are faced by both large-scale and small-scale poultry farmers; nevertheless, smaller companies are typically more susceptible to experiences of financial distress. Integrated poultry operations, which include breeding, production, and processing, have the potential to suffer losses across a number of different segments.

Government Response Costs

Governments frequently develop compensation programmes for farmers who have been negatively impacted, which results in increased financial constraints for the farmers. Governments make investments in research, monitoring, and preventative measures, which contribute to overall public spending. These investments are referred to as "investments in prevention."

Insurance and risk management

When it comes to avian influenza, insurance coverage may have certain restrictions, and compensation may not be sufficient to cover all of the monetary losses that have been sustained. The implementation of risk mitigation tactics, such as biosecurity controls and contingency planning, is becoming increasingly common among poultry producing companies.

The global impact on prices

The occurrence of outbreaks of avian influenza is a factor that contributes to price volatility in chicken products around the world. Uncertainty in the market

can cause volatility in prices, which can have an effect on both consumers and producers.

The long-term resilience of the industry

Restoring the faith of consumers and the market is a task that the chicken business will face for a considerable amount of time after an outbreak. In order to maintain the industry's resilience, it is necessary to make continuous investments in biosecurity measures and research in order to forestall such outbreaks in the future.

International Cooperation

When it comes to surveillance, reporting, and coordinated responses, international cooperation is required since avian influenza is a worldwide problem that requires global attention. In order to gain a more comprehensive understanding of the virus and to develop more efficient methods of control, collaborative research activities are essential.

Public Perception and Communication

Transparency and communication are discussed here. When it comes to controlling public opinion and

preserving trust, transparent communication from authorities and influential players in the sector is absolutely necessary. Consumer education is the following: It is essential to educate customers on the safety measures that are currently in place as well as the impact that outbreaks have on food safety.

It is necessary to take a holistic approach that involves industry stakeholders, government, and global collaboration in order to successfully navigate the economic ramifications of outbreaks of avian influenza. It is vital to make consistent investments in research, biosecurity measures, and risk management tactics in order to construct resilience and maintain a poultry sector that is both robust and secure.

Health Implications for Humans

Zoonotic Potential: Understanding Human Transmission

In the context of public health and disease prevention, the zoonotic potential of avian influenza, in particular subtypes such as H5N1 and H7N9, is an essential component. When it comes to surveillance, preventive, and preparedness activities, having a solid understanding of how the virus might be transmitted from birds to humans is absolutely necessary.

Zoonotic Transmission Pathways

1. Direct Contact: The most common way for humans to become infected is through direct contact with diseased birds or the settings in which they live. Individuals who work in environments where they come into contact with diseased birds, such as those seen in live bird markets or backyard farming, are at a greater risk of contracting the disease.

2. Transmission within the Air: There is evidence that avian influenza can be transmitted to humans through the air, despite the fact that it is largely a respiratory virus that affects birds. There is a risk of inhaling respiratory droplets that contain the virus for individuals who are in close proximity to infected birds.

3. Zoonotic Strains: Because of its high pathogenicity in birds and its capacity to cause serious sickness and death in people, the *H5N1* strain has been the subject of a substantial amount of attention. Another zoonotic strain, *H7N9*, has shown that it is capable of infecting humans. Cases of human illness have been linked to interactions with live poultry.

4. Virus Receptor Binding Specificity: The process by which the virus is able to recognize human cell receptors is an essential step in the process of effectively transmitting the virus to humans - Human Receptor Binding. The compatibility of the virus with human receptors is a factor that plays a role in determining whether or not it is able to transcend the species barrier.

5. Genetic reassortment: This occurs when human-adapted strains of influenza viruses swap genetic

material with avian influenza viruses, is an important element in the transmission of influenza from one species to another. The emergence of novel strains that have the potential to cause pandemics can be a consequence of this process.

Risk Factors for Human Transmission and Transmission

- Occupational Exposure: People who work in the poultry sector, from farmers to market workers, are at a greater risk of contracting respiratory illnesses because of their close contact with live birds.
- Surveillance and Early Detection: It is essential to conduct surveillance in high-risk areas and to discover outbreaks as soon as possible in order to reduce the number of people who are exposed to the disease.

*The following are examples of clinical manifestations
in humans:*

- Symptoms of the Respiratory System: Avian
  influenza has the potential to produce severe
  respiratory symptoms in humans, such as
  pneumonia and acute respiratory distress
  syndrome (ARDS).
- Significantly High Mortality Rates: It has been
  found that certain strains, like as H5N1, are
  connected with significant fatality rates in
  human infections.

Global Surveillance and Reporting

For the purpose of monitoring avian influenza and
identifying potential zoonotic outbreaks, global
surveillance networks and international cooperation
between nations are absolutely necessary. Providing
timely reports of human instances and sharing
information in an open and honest manner are also
essential components of coordinated responses.

Preventive Measures

- Biosecurity Measures: There is a reduction in the risk of avian influenza being transmitted to people when poultry farms use strong biosecurity measures.
- Programs of Vaccination: Vaccination programs in poultry, when they are practicable, contribute to a reduction in the prevalence of the virus across the poultry population.

Preparation for Pandemics

- Antiviral Development: The development of antiviral drugs that are effective against strains of avian influenza is a crucial component of pandemic preparedness.
- Vaccine Development: Aiming to develop vaccinations that are effective against future pandemic strains, ongoing research in the field of vaccine development is now underway.
- Education and Awareness of the Community: When it comes to teaching the general people about the dangers of avian influenza and the preventative actions that may be taken,

community awareness initiatives and public health messages play an extremely important role.

The rapid reporting of suspected cases is an important factor in early intervention and containment; therefore, it is important to encourage prompt reporting of suspected cases.

A comprehensive approach that encompasses surveillance, research, preventative measures, and worldwide collaboration is required in order to gain an understanding of the zoonotic potential of avian influenza. Through the implementation of these components, public health systems have the potential to improve their capacity to identify and respond to possible risks, hence reducing the likelihood of human transmission and the possibility of pandemics.

Pandemic Preparedness: Lessons from Bird Flu for Global Health

The emergence and transmission of avian influenza, more usually referred to as bird flu, have supplied important lessons that are essential for the preparation of the global pandemic. When these lessons are analyzed, public health systems, policymakers, and the international community are provided with insights that may be used to improve surveillance, response mechanisms, and collaboration in the face of possible pandemics.

Interconnection of Human, Animal, and Environmental Health

The bird flu outbreaks underline the relevance of the One Health approach, emphasizing the interconnection of human, animal, and environmental health. Diseases such as avian influenza bring to light the fact that health concerns are not limited to a single species and require a response that is collaborative and takes into account multiple sectors.

Early Detection and Reporting

Timely Surveillance: Early detection is essential for avoiding the spread of outbreaks and stopping them from becoming more severe. In order to effectively discover potential dangers in a timely manner, surveillance systems need to be sturdy, transparent, and capable of doing so.

In order to contribute to a coordinated global response, it is important to encourage governments to swiftly report and coordinate information regarding emerging illnesses.

Genetic Reassortment and Strain Evolution

Avian influenza's ability to undergo genetic reassortment underscores the flexibility of influenza viruses. It is necessary to maintain vigilance in order to monitor alterations in the virus that have the potential to impart pandemic potential. For this reason, continual research and surveillance activities are essential.

Zoonotic Threats and Animal Reservoirs

Understanding Zoonotic Risks: The zoonotic potential of avian influenza underscores the need to study and monitor diseases at the human-animal interface. The significance of surveillance in these populations is brought to light by the recognition of the function that wildlife, particularly wild birds, play as potential reservoirs.

Communication of Dangers and Awareness of the Environment

In order to establish public trust and encourage compliance with preventive measures, it is essential for health authorities to communicate in a clear and open manner. Involving communities in the process of understanding the dangers and preventative actions increases collective resilience.

Poultry Industry Biosecurity

Lessons from avian influenza outbreaks emphasize the need for stringent biosecurity measures in the poultry industry. Also, vaccination programs in poultry, where feasible, contribute to reducing the prevalence of avian influenza strains.

Vaccination Development for Humans

The urgency of avian influenza outbreaks highlights the necessity for continued funding in research for vaccinations effective against future pandemic strains and also ensuring that vaccines are accessible on a

worldwide scale is essential for achieving equitable pandemic response and containment.

Antiviral Medications and Treatment Protocols

Availability of Antivirals: The development and maintenance of a supply of antiviral medications that are effective against avian influenza strains is a factor that contributes to treatment and prevention efforts. The establishment of treatment procedures for severe instances assists healthcare systems in managing the impact of the disease on human populations.

International Collaboration and Coordination

Collaborative efforts, exemplified by global surveillance networks like the World Health Organization's Global Influenza Surveillance and Response System, enhance preparedness. Establishing rapid response mechanisms at the international level facilitates the coordinated deployment of resources during a pandemic.

Community Health Infrastructure

Strengthening Health Systems: In order to effectively prepare for and respond to pandemics, it is essential to strengthen both local and national health systems. Increasing the capabilities of healthcare professionals and institutions is essential to ensuring a strong frontline fight against newly emerging infectious illnesses.

Research and Innovation

It is vital to conduct ongoing research and innovation in order to adjust strategies to the ever-changing nature of influenza viruses. Utilizing technology breakthroughs allows for improvements to be made in the areas of diagnosis, surveillance, and treatment modalities.

Global Governance and Policy Coordination

A cohesive response to pandemics can be ensured by international collaboration in the development of coordinated policies and tactics. Minimizing uncertainty and facilitating a unified global response can be accomplished by harmonizing policies pertaining to travel, trade, and public health measures.

Adaptive Learning and Knowledge Sharing

An adaptive learning approach, informed by experiences like bird flu outbreaks, ensures that responses evolve with emerging challenges. Increasing global pandemic resilience can be accomplished through the establishment of platforms that facilitate the sharing of knowledge and practises that have proven to be effective.

The lessons that may be learned from epidemics of bird flu are extremely helpful when it comes to developing a proactive and adaptable strategy for pandemic preparedness. Incorporating these lessons into global health policies and practices will be essential for protecting public health and ensuring a coordinated and effective response to future pandemics. This is because the globe is currently facing a variety of health risks that are constantly evolving.

Detection and Diagnosis

Surveillance Methods: Monitoring Avian Influenza in Birds

Surveillance techniques are extremely important in the process of monitoring avian influenza in birds because they allow for the early detection of the disease, the

evaluation of risk factors, and the prompt deployment of control measures. Considering the varied characteristics of avian influenza viruses and the possible influence they could have on the health of both animals and humans, it is necessary to implement comprehensive surveillance strategies that cover both wild and domestic bird populations. The purpose of this article is to investigate the wide variety of surveillance techniques that are utilized in order to keep track of and comprehend the dynamics of avian influenza.

Wild Bird Surveillance

Sampling in wild birds is a common practice in the field of surveillance. This is because migratory routes are places where avian influenza viruses can be introduced or propagated. The collection of environmental samples, which includes the collection of water from wild bird habitats and other environmental sources, is an effective method for determining whether or not the virus is present in certain environments.

Domestic Poultry Surveillance

The routine monitoring that takes place within domestic poultry farms includes the testing of samples taken from live birds, as well as swabs taken from surfaces and equipment. The establishment of sentinel flocks, which are regularly watched for indicators of illness, improves the early diagnosis of illnesses inside commercial poultry farms.

Serological Testing

Serological tests are used to identify antibodies that are created as a result of exposure to the avian influenza virus. The surveillance of subclinical infections includes the following: Through the use of serological testing, subclinical infections in bird populations can be identified, which contributes to the early intervention process.

Virological Testing

Polymerase Chain Reaction (PCR) and Reverse Transcription Polymerase Chain Reaction (RT-PCR) are molecular methods used to detect viral RNA in samples. Culturing and isolating the virus from samples provide definitive proof of active infection.

Genetic Sequencing

Genomic Analysis: Genetic sequencing of avian influenza viruses provides insights into their genetic makeup, helping identify strains and track their evolution.

Identification of High-Risk Variants: Sequencing assists in identifying genetic changes associated with increased pathogenicity or zoonotic potential

Real-Time Surveillance Networks

Global Influenza Surveillance Networks: Global networks, like the World Health Organization's Global Influenza Surveillance and Response System, facilitate real-time information exchange and coordinated responses.

Data Sharing: Timely sharing of surveillance data between countries enhances collective preparedness and response efforts.

Wildlife Reservoir Surveillance

Surveillance in wildlife reservoirs, especially waterfowl, contributes to understanding the prevalence and dynamics of avian influenza in these populations. Studying interactions between wild birds and domestic poultry informs the assessment of interspecies transmission risks.

Syndromic Surveillance

Syndromic surveillance involves monitoring clinical signs of avian influenza in birds, such as respiratory distress or changes in behavior. Syndromic surveillance supports early warning systems for outbreaks in domestic poultry and wild bird populations.

Community-Based Surveillance

Community-based surveillance engages local communities in reporting unusual bird deaths or signs of illness. Rapid reporting from communities enhances early detection and response efforts.

Serological Surveys in Humans

Surveillance also extends to monitoring human populations for serological evidence of exposure to avian influenza viruses. Identifying individuals with antibodies to avian influenza viruses helps detect potential zoonotic events.

Integration of Data Sources

Integrating data from various sources, including virological, serological, and environmental data, enhances the comprehensive understanding of avian influenza dynamics. Data integration supports predictive modeling to anticipate potential outbreaks and guide preemptive interventions.

Capacity Building and Training

Capacity building initiatives focus on enhancing the skills of professionals involved in surveillance, ensuring accurate sample collection, testing, and data interpretation. Training programs raise awareness about the importance of surveillance among stakeholders, including veterinarians, farmers, and wildlife conservationists.

Global Collaboration and Reporting Protocols

Standardized reporting protocols enhance consistency in surveillance data reporting across countries. Collaborative efforts in surveillance, guided by international organizations, promote a unified response to global avian influenza threats.

Investment in Research and Technology

Ongoing investment in research and technology development ensures the integration of cutting-edge tools in avian influenza surveillance.

Innovation in Detection Methods

Innovation in detection methods, such as the development of rapid diagnostic tests, improves the efficiency of surveillance programs.

Using a combination of conventional and cutting-edge surveillance techniques, the comprehensive approach to monitoring avian influenza in birds is known as the multifaceted approach. It is vital to include these methods into a worldwide framework of collaboration, information exchange, and adaptive measures in order to stay ahead of the ever-changing nature of avian influenza viruses and to minimize the impact that these viruses have on the health of both animals and humans.

Human Diagnosis: Identifying and Confirming Cases

The identification of avian influenza in human beings is an essential component of public health surveillance, since it enables prompt action and the implementation of containment measures simultaneously. Clinical evaluation, laboratory testing, and epidemiological studies are all components that are utilized in the process of identifying and validating cases. The purpose of this article is to examine the comprehensive process of diagnosing avian influenza in people, focusing on the intricacies and difficulties connected with proper case identification.

Clinical Presentation

Avian influenza often presents with severe respiratory symptoms, including cough, difficulty breathing, and pneumonia. Fever, malaise, and systemic symptoms may also be present, resembling symptoms of other respiratory illnesses.

Epidemiological Context

Gathering a detailed history of the patient's exposure, including recent travel to areas with avian influenza outbreaks or contact with birds, is crucial. Identifying occupational risk, such as working in the poultry industry, helps assess potential exposure.

Clinical Assessment

A thorough physical examination, focusing on respiratory signs and symptoms, guides clinical assessment. Chest imaging, including X-rays and computed tomography (CT) scans, aids in evaluating the extent of respiratory involvement.

Laboratory Testing

Molecular testing, such as PCR, is employed to detect viral RNA in respiratory samples. Culturing the virus from clinical specimens provides definitive confirmation of avian influenza infection. Serological tests detect antibodies produced in response to the virus, aiding in retrospective diagnosis.

Genetic Sequencing

Genetic sequencing helps identify the specific strain of avian influenza virus, contributing to surveillance and understanding of transmission dynamics. Sequencing assists in identifying genetic changes that may confer increased pathogenicity or potential for human-to-human transmission.

Rapid Diagnostic Tests

Rapid diagnostic tests designed for point-of-care use provide quick results, facilitating timely decision-making in healthcare settings. Some tests detect viral antigens directly, offering a rapid means of confirming infection.

Serological Surveys

Serological surveys in human populations help identify individuals with previous exposure to avian influenza viruses. Studying seroprevalence provides insights into population immunity and potential risks of future outbreaks.

Differential Diagnosis

Given the similarity of avian influenza symptoms to other respiratory illnesses, a thorough differential diagnosis is essential. Distinguishing avian influenza from seasonal influenza strains is critical for appropriate treatment and public health measures.

Case Definitions and Reporting Protocols

Establishing standardized case definitions ensures consistency in identifying and reporting avian influenza cases. Timely reporting of suspected cases to health authorities facilitates rapid response and containment efforts.

Collaboration with Animal Health Authorities

Collaboration between human and animal health authorities, following the One Health approach, helps identify and address potential sources of infection. Monitoring avian influenza in animal populations provides early warning for potential human cases.

Surveillance of Close Contacts

Identifying and monitoring close contacts of confirmed cases is crucial for preventing secondary transmission. Implementing quarantine measures for contacts, especially those with symptoms, reduces the risk of further spread.

Public Health Messaging and Education

Public health messaging and education campaigns raise awareness about avian influenza symptoms and the importance of seeking medical attention. Encouraging the public to report suspected cases promptly contributes to early detection.

Antiviral Treatment

Antiviral medications, such as neuraminidase inhibitors, are initiated early in confirmed cases to reduce severity and duration of illness. Establishing treatment protocols ensures consistency in the clinical management of avian influenza cases.

Hospital Preparedness

Hospitals implement strict infection control measures to prevent nosocomial transmission. Designated isolation units help manage and treat confirmed cases while minimizing the risk of exposure to healthcare workers and other patients.

Global Reporting and Collaboration

Countries follow international reporting protocols to share information about confirmed avian influenza cases. Global collaboration enhances the collective understanding of avian influenza and supports coordinated responses.

Research for Therapeutics and Vaccines

Ongoing research explores novel therapeutics effective against avian influenza viruses. Development of vaccines targeting potential pandemic strains remains a priority for global health preparedness.

Surveillance Beyond Confirmed Cases

Ongoing syndromic surveillance monitors respiratory illness patterns to detect potential outbreaks even before confirmed cases arise. Continued surveillance in wildlife populations contributes to understanding the ongoing risk of zoonotic transmission.

Community Engagement in Surveillance

Engaging communities in surveillance efforts encourages active participation in reporting unusual bird deaths or human cases. Community involvement builds trust and enhances the effectiveness of surveillance programs.

The process of diagnosing avian influenza in people requires a multi-pronged approach that incorporates clinical evaluation, laboratory testing, and epidemiological research. Considering the complications involved in distinguishing avian influenza from other respiratory infections and the possibility of zoonotic transmission, it is imperative that continued research be conducted, international collaboration be established, and a proactive One Health approach be taken to ensure the safety of global health.

Prevention and Control Strategies

Vaccination: Protecting Birds and Humans

Vaccination plays a crucial role in preserving both bird and human populations against the threat of avian influenza. It is necessary to make vaccination efforts that are both strategic and targeted because of the complicated dynamics of avian influenza viruses. These viruses have the ability to cause serious disease in both wild and farmed birds, and they can also occasionally become infectious to people. In this article, we explore into the vast landscape of avian influenza vaccine, discussing its accomplishments and problems, as well as the twin goal of preserving the health of both humans and birds.

Avian Influenza Vaccines for Birds

Various types of avian influenza vaccinations are utilized in poultry, including *inactivated vaccines*, *live attenuated vaccines*, and *vector vaccines*. In many cases, vaccines are created to target particular strains that are predominant in a particular region.

Preventive Vaccination in Poultry

- Broiler and Layer hens: Broiler and layer hens are given vaccinations on a regular basis in order to avoid the spread of avian influenza and to limit economic losses.
- Breeder Flocks: The vaccination of breeder flocks helps to increase the number of chicks that are born with maternal antibodies, which provides early protection.

Mass Vaccination Campaigns

- Routine Vaccination: Many countries employ regular vaccination programs, particularly in regions that have prior experience with outbreaks of avian influenza.
- Emergency Response Vaccination: In response to outbreaks, mass vaccination campaigns may be initiated to control the spread of the virus.

Challenges in Poultry Vaccination

- Matching Vaccine Strains: Adapting vaccines to match circulating strains is a challenge due to the genetic diversity of avian influenza viruses.
- Vaccine Coverage: Ensuring comprehensive vaccine coverage across poultry populations, including backyard and free-ranging birds, can be logistically challenging.

Surveillance in Vaccinated Flocks

Surveillance is vital in order to evaluate the efficacy of vaccination programs and identify any infections that have not yet been eradicated. Surveillance works to identify new variants that may be able to circumvent the immunity that is provided by the vaccinations that are already available.

Wild Bird Vaccination Considerations

Vaccinating wild bird populations is difficult because of the abundance of habitats that they inhabit, which are frequently inaccessible. Given the close closeness of domestic poultry to humans and the economic implications of outbreaks, the primary focus of vaccination efforts is on domestic poultry.

Zoonotic Potential and Human Vaccination

Vaccination of domestic poultry contributes, in a roundabout way, to lowering the risk of infection that is transmitted from animals to humans.

Preventative measures against future pandemic strains are the goal of research into human vaccinations, which is being conducted with the intention of developing human vaccines.

Challenges in Human Vaccine Development

The rapid evolution of avian influenza viruses poses challenges in developing human vaccines that provide broad protection. Antigenic drift and shift necessitate continuous surveillance to identify strains for inclusion in human vaccine formulations.

Pandemic Preparedness

Certain nations have stockpiles of pre-pandemic vaccines that are aimed at avian influenza viruses that have the potential to cause a pandemic.

The acceleration of vaccine development timelines in the case of a pandemic danger is the primary focus of ongoing research.

Adjuvants and Vaccine Efficacy

Adjuvants are used to enhance the immune response to avian influenza vaccines, improving their efficacy. Selection of appropriate adjuvants is crucial, considering the diversity of avian influenza strains.

Education and Outreach

Educating poultry farmers on the need of vaccination and biosecurity measures is crucial for the effectiveness of avian influenza control initiatives. Vaccination is emphasized as an important factor in reducing bird flu and potential human infections in public awareness efforts.

Vaccination against avian influenza, which can be administered to both birds and humans, is an essential component of the worldwide effort to reduce the effect of this multifaceted and ever-evolving virus. In order to keep ahead of the problems posed by avian influenza and to protect both animal and human populations all over the world, it is essential to integrate cutting-edge technologies, insights gained from surveillance, and international collaboration.

Biosecurity Measures: Containing the Spread

In order to prevent the spread of avian influenza, which is a highly contagious virus that poses considerable hazards to the health of both poultry and humans, it is essential to implement biosecurity measures that are particularly effective. Through the implementation of comprehensive biosecurity procedures, it is vital to avoid the entry of avian influenza viruses and to minimize the spread of these viruses whenever possible.

Farm Entry Protocols

Restricting access to poultry farms helps control the entry of potential sources of avian influenza. Farm personnel and visitors undergo changes in footwear and clothing to minimize the risk of introducing the virus.

Separation of Poultry Flocks

Creating isolated areas for different poultry flocks helps prevent direct and indirect contact, reducing the risk of virus transmission. Well-designed facilities with separate pens and biosecurity zones contribute to effective separation.

Wildlife Management

The utilization of avian deterrents, which include scare devices and nets, serves to reduce the amount of contact that occurs between wild birds and poultry. The risk of introduction is decreased when water supplies are protected from contamination by wild birds.

Quarantine measures

Implementing quarantine measures for newly arrival birds enables for observation and testing before integrating them into current flocks. During the period of quarantine, it is important to perform regular health checks in order to identify any possible early indicators of avian influenza.

Strict Hygiene methods

The implementation of stringent handwashing and disinfection methods helps to limit the likelihood that personnel may transmit the virus. Sanitizing tools, cars, and equipment on a regular basis reduces the likelihood that fomite will be transmitted from one person to another.

Pest Control

Keeping rodents and insects under control helps to guarantee that they do not operate as vectors for the spread of avian influenza. The correct storage of feed helps to prevent contamination and minimizes the likelihood that pests will be drawn to the area.

Surveillance Programs

The purpose of surveillance is to detect the presence of avian influenza by conducting regular testing on poultry flocks. The monitoring of wild bird populations is an extension of surveillance that is used to identify potential sources of infection.

Emergency Response Plans

Having well-defined emergency response plans enables rapid deployment of measures in the event of an outbreak. Clear communication protocols ensure efficient coordination among stakeholders during emergencies.

Culling Protocols

The removal of diseased or exposed birds from the population as quickly as possible is an essential biosecurity step that helps to prevent the disease from spreading further. The proper disposal procedures for culled birds, which may include safe burial or incineration, are an essential component of containment efforts.

Vaccination Programs

Vaccination, when as part of a biosecurity strategy, contributes to reducing the occurrence of avian influenza as well as the severity of the disease. The effectiveness of vaccination programs can be improved by ensuring that all vaccines are covered and that compliance is maintained.

Personal Protective Equipment (PPE)

Personnel working with poultry, particularly during outbreaks, are required to use suitable PPE in order to prevent direct contact with diseased birds. The danger of personnel becoming carriers of the virus is mitigated by the use of biosecure clothing and footwear designated specifically for that purpose.

Traceability Systems

Keeping complete records of bird movements, interactions, and interventions** is an important part of supporting traceability during outbreaks. In the event of an outbreak, digital traceability solutions improve the speed and accuracy of information sharing, which improves the overall situation.

Global Governance and Information Sharing

Global governance systems make it possible to share information, coordinate responses, and work together to prevent the spread of avian influenza. Information that is shared in a timely manner guarantees that a collective and prompt reaction can be provided to emergent outbreaks.

Integration with One Health Approach

Recognizing the interconnection of human, animal, and environmental health is accomplished by aligning biosecurity measures together with the One Health approach. The efficiency of biosecurity initiatives is improved when there is collaboration between the health, agricultural, and environmental sectors.

The foundation of efforts to restrict the spread of avian influenza is the implementation of biosecurity measures, which protects both the welfare of animals and the health of the general people. In order to mitigate the dangers associated with outbreaks of avian influenza and to ensure a resilient response to future difficulties, it is necessary that these strategies be continuously refined and adopted on a worldwide scale.

Global Cooperation: International Efforts in Combating Bird Flu

As a result of the fact that avian influenza, often known as bird flu, poses a global threat to the health of both humans and animals, it is necessary for international organizations to work together to combat this disease. For the purpose of preventing outbreaks, managing the spread of the virus, and mitigating the potential for zoonotic transmission, the fight against bird flu involves coordinated efforts, the sharing of information, and joint activities.

There are international organizations and alliances, such as the World Health Organization (WHO), which includes: Through the provision of guidelines and the facilitation of collaboration between member nations, the World Health Organization (WHO) plays a pivotal role in the coordination of worldwide responses against bird flu.

A statement from the Food and Agriculture Organization (FAO): Through the provision of expertise in animal health, the promotion of sustainable farming practices, and the support of capacity building, the Food and Agriculture Organization (FAO) contributes to global initiatives.

The World Organisation for Animal Health (OIE) is the intergovernmental body that is responsible for animal health. The OIE is responsible for establishing international standards and guidelines for the prevention and control of avian influenza.

Global Influenza Surveillance Networks: Collaborative networks, such as the Global Influenza Surveillance and Response System, make it possible to monitor avian influenza strains in real time and share information with one another.

International initiatives entail the development and refinement of predictive models in order to foresee probable outbreaks and inform preparedness measures. These models are referred to as pandemic prediction models.

Joint Research Initiatives: Countries and research institutes engage in exchanging genetic data of avian influenza viruses, aiding in the discovery of new strains.

The development of vaccines is the primary focus of international research partnerships, with the goal of creating vaccines that provide comprehensive protection against a wide variety of avian influenza bacteria.

Surveillance and Reporting Protocols: Standardized Surveillance Protocols: The adoption of standardized surveillance protocols is made possible by international collaboration, which improves the consistency and comparability of different data sets.

Rapid Reporting Systems: The timely reporting of cases of avian influenza to international organizations makes it easier to respond in a timely and coordinated manner.

Capacity Building and Training.

Training Programs: International organizations offer training programs to increase the capacity of veterinarians, healthcare professionals, and policymakers in dealing with avian influenza.

In the realm of knowledge transfer, exchange programs and efforts that promote knowledge sharing contribute to the development of a worldwide workforce that is capable of addressing issues posed by bird flu.

Cross-Border Cooperation

Regional Alliances: Countries that are located within specific regions come together to create alliances in order to improve collective responses, share resources, and coordinate control measures.

Exchange of Information: In order to prevent the spread of avian influenza across international borders, cross-border cooperation comprises the exchange of information regarding outbreaks, surveillance results, and control tactics concerning the disease.

One Health Approach

Interdisciplinary Collaboration: The implementation of the One Health approach places an emphasis on interdisciplinary collaboration between the human, animal, and environmental health sectors.

Cooperation in the Formulation of Policies: The establishment of cooperative policies that acknowledge the interconnectivity of health systems is an important part of international initiatives.

Emergency Response Coordination

Rapid Response Teams: Countries that are experiencing outbreaks of avian influenza are assisted by international organizations that coordinate the deployment of quick response teams.

Mobilization of Resources: In order to provide assistance to regions that have been impacted, collaborative activities require the mobilization of resources such as manpower, equipment, and other forms of financial help.

International Conferences and Forums

Global Summits: Convening global summits and conferences gives a venue for countries to exchange their experiences, discuss issues, and strategize on their collective measures against bird flu.

Scientific Exchanges: International forums create an environment that is conducive to scientific exchanges, which in turn encourages innovation and the development of control mechanisms that are very successful.

Technology Transfer

Sharing Diagnostic technology: Advanced nations work together to share diagnostic technology with regions that have limited resources. This allows for the identification of avian influenza cases to be completed more quickly and with more precision.

Telemedicine projects: Technology transfer includes telemedicine projects, which connect specialists with frontline healthcare workers in regions that are experiencing outbreaks.

Legal Frameworks and Treaties

Countries take part in international treaties and agreements that establish obligations and commitments in the event of avian influenza outbreaks. These treaties and agreements are referred to as international treaties.

Harmonisation of regulations: Efforts are being undertaken to ensure that a unified global response is achieved by harmonising rules that are connected to the control and prevention of avian influenza.

Information Sharing Platforms

Worldwide Databases: Establishing worldwide databases improves the sharing of information on avian influenza strains, outbreaks, and control actions.

Real-Time Communication: Platforms for information sharing make it possible to communicate in real time during times of emergency, which speeds up the response time.

Crisis Diplomacy

Diplomatic Channels: Diplomatic channels are deployed for the purpose of crisis diplomacy, which aims to encourage collaboration between nations and handle geopolitical concerns that may have an impact on efforts to control avian influenza.

Joint statements: Countries send out joint statements in which they vow to working together to take action in response to new dangers.

A collaborative commitment to shared duties, mutual assistance, and the realization that the global community is interconnected in the face of health hazards are essential to the success of international efforts to battle bird flu. In order to build resilience and ensure a coordinated response to the ever-changing challenges posed by avian influenza, it is of the utmost importance that governments, international organizations, and stakeholders continue to work together.

Overcoming Challenges

Communication Strategies: Public Awareness and Education

When it comes to teaching communities and boosting public awareness about avian influenza, also known as bird flu, effective communication tactics are absolutely necessary. When it comes to preventing outbreaks, ensuring early reporting, and encouraging a coordinated response, it is essential to promote understanding of the dangers, preventative measures, and the role that everyone can play.

Clear and Accessible Messaging

The utilization of language that is both clear and simple in messaging guarantees that information is accessible to a wide audience, including individuals with varied levels of education. Providing material in a variety of languages allows awareness campaigns to be more inclusive and cater to a wider range of populations.

Targeted Outreach

Increasing the relevance and effectiveness of communications by adapting them for different demographic groups, such as farmers, healthcare workers, and the general public, is an effective strategy. Understanding the local contexts and customs is helpful in tailoring communication tactics to the distinct requirements and concerns of various communities. This type of communication is referred to as "community-specific communication."

Multi-Channel Approach

Utilizing a combination of traditional and digital media, such as television, radio, social media, and print, is an effective way to optimize both reach and engagement. Establishing partnerships with influential members of the community and powerful figures in the community can significantly boost the credibility and efficiency of communication efforts.

Visual Communication

The incorporation of infographics and visual aids simplifies complicated material, making it simpler for the general audience to understand important concepts. Creating videos that are educational helps to transmit important messages and instructions in a style that is interesting to the audience.

Public Service Announcements (PSAs)

PSAs provide messages that are both succinct and impactful, thereby increasing awareness without overwhelming the audience. Public service announcements (PSAs) that are broadcast on television, radio, and online platforms have a wider audience and are more likely to be widely disseminated.

Interactive Educational Programs

The facilitation of interactive learning experiences, which include the provision of opportunities for questions and clarifications, is made possible through the conduct of workshops and webinars at educational institutions. When teaching about avian influenza is incorporated into the curriculum of schools, it gives students the opportunity to become aware of the disease at a young age and encourages them to share their knowledge with their families.

Engagement with Local Communities

The holding of community meetings encourages direct interaction, which enables the exchange of information and concerns that are specific to the community. Campaigns that go door-to-door with informative materials ensure that even underserved or rural communities receive vital information.

Storytelling and Narratives

The act of sharing personal experiences of persons who have been touched by avian influenza humanizes the issue and makes it more relatable to the general audience. Inspiring others to follow in the footsteps of communities that have successfully implemented preventive measures are accomplished by highlighting the success stories of communities that have successfully implemented these measures.

Question and Answer Sessions

The public is able to seek clarity on specific concerns by participating in live question and answer sessions, which can be held either in-person or online. Involving specialists in avian influenza in question and answer sessions helps to develop trust and credibility in the information that is being delivered.

Emergency Communication Systems

Establishing hotlines for the purpose of reporting suspicious cases or seeking information guarantees that communication channels are both direct and immediate. It is possible to reach a large number of people, including those who do not have access to the internet, by sending text message notifications about updates and preventative steps about avian influenza.

Social Media Campaigns

The creation and promotion of specific hashtags assists in the organizing of information and motivates users of social media to engage within the campaign. Increasing the shareability of content on social media platforms can be accomplished through the utilization of visuals, such as infographics and brief movies.

Partnerships with Educational Institutions

Working together with educational institutions, such as schools and universities, to incorporate teaching about avian influenza into relevant curricula ensures that the impact will be both long-lasting and extensive. Giving students the opportunity to participate in projects that raise awareness about avian influenza gives them the ability to act as ambassadors for furthering the dissemination of information within their communities.

Public Demonstrations and Simulations

The act of conducting live demonstrations of preventive measures, such as the correct way to wash one's hands and the practices of biosecurity, helps to reinforce learning. Communities are better prepared to deal with potential outbreaks when they participate in simulation drills that are organized to enhance their readiness to respond to emergency situations.

Crisis Communication Planning

Creating and spreading preparedness messaging in advance ensures that the general public is informed and adequately prepared to respond in the event of an outbreak. Communicating clear reporting procedures for suspected situations guarantees that the general public is aware of how and where to seek assistance.

Incorporating Cultural Sensitivity

Tailoring communication to respect cultural beliefs and customs helps to reduce opposition and more effectively promotes adoption of preventative actions. There is a correlation between the incorporation of avian influenza education into cultural events and festivals and an increase in the level of involvement and participation.

Regular Updates and Information Dissemination

In order to keep the public aware of the ongoing issue, it is important to provide regular updates on the present situation, preventative actions, and any changes in guidelines. In order to ensure that the general public has easy access to information that is both accurate and up to date, centralized internet platforms should be established.

Governmental and Non-Governmental Collaboration

When governments work together with non-governmental groups and international agencies, they are able to build a unified front in the process of disseminating information. When resources and knowledge are pooled together, it is possible to conduct communication campaigns that are more thorough and have a greater reach with shared resources.

Feedback Mechanisms

The collection of feedback through the use of surveys and feedback forms will allow for the ongoing improvement of communication tactics. Adapting communication strategies based on public reaction ensures that communications are successful and resonate with the audience that is being targeted.

Celebrity Endorsements for Advocacy

Involving celebrities as advocates for avian influenza awareness attracts attention to the cause and leverages each celebrity's power for the purpose of conveying positive messages. Celebrities who take part in public service campaigns contribute to improved visibility and interaction with the public.

Integration with Other Health initiatives

Creating synergy and making the most of resources is accomplished by integrating avian influenza awareness with larger health initiatives. The One Health method is strengthened by putting an emphasis on the interdependence of human and animal health.

When it comes to empowering communities to protect themselves and preventing the spread of avian influenza, comprehensive communication techniques play a vital part in the process. Public awareness and education become important weapons in the global effort to limit the hazards associated with bird flu outbreaks when they are communicated in a way that is clear, targeted, and sensitive to cultural norms.

Ethical Considerations: Balancing Health and Animal Welfare

In order to effectively manage avian influenza, it is necessary to navigate a more complicated ethical terrain, one in which the health of both humans and animals is at stake. The difficulties that arise from attempting to strike a balance between safeguarding public health, providing food security, and protecting the welfare of birds are particularly complex.

Preventive Measures and Animal Welfare

The implementation of biosecurity measures to prevent the transmission of avian influenza may require restrictive measures regarding the movement and social contact of birds. When it comes to maintaining the birds' well-being, ethical considerations include reducing the amount of stress they experience during increased biosecurity measures.

Culling and Euthanasia

It is frequently essential to cull birds that have been exposed to or infected with a disease in order to successfully control the disease and prevent its further spread. The adoption of compassionate euthanasia techniques is required by ethical concerns in order to reduce the amount of suffering that occurs during culling operations.

Economic Impact on farms

Culling procedures can have major economic implications for poultry farms. Considerations about livelihoods are also important. The provision of just compensation and support to farmers who have been adversely affected in order to reduce the amount of economic damage they have suffered is an example of an ethical practice.

Transparent Communication

The public's trust can be increased by transparent communication regarding the necessity of control measures. The goal of ethical communication is to strike a balance between eliminating unneeded alarm or stigmatization and maintaining transparency.

Human Health and Zoonotic Risks

The measures that are taken to manage avian influenza are designed to protect human health by preventing the spread of the virus from animals to humans.

When it comes to research and monitoring, ethical research and monitoring activities are centered on gaining an understanding of the hazards of zoonotic transmission and finding ways to mitigate those risks.

Vaccination Strategies

Although vaccination is an essential method for combating avian influenza, there are ethical considerations that must be taken into account when administering it. Immunization tactics that adhere to ethical standards put an emphasis on the effectiveness of vaccines while also monitoring and decreasing the risk of adverse effects.

Animal Welfare Standards

Ethical management requires a commitment to adhering to the standards that have been developed for animal welfare. Efforts are undertaken to continuously enhance animal welfare procedures while adhering to the limits of disease control techniques.

Local and Global Equity

Ethical concerns include making certain that control measures, resources, and assistance are allocated in an equitable manner, that is, both locally and worldwide. Recognizing that avian influenza is a problem that affects everyone on the planet, collaborative efforts respect the values of global solidarity.

Long-Term Sustainability

Ethical management of avian influenza takes into consideration the influence that control measures have on the environment. In order to achieve long-term sustainability, it is necessary to strike a balance between the urgent needs for disease control and the more general ecological factors.

Community Involvement and Consultation

Informed Decision-Making: Ethical practices require communicating with impacted communities and stakeholders to ensure that their input is included in the decision-making process. The dissemination of information to communities assists in the development of an understanding and acceptance of control measures.

Emergency Response Ethics

Ethical emergency responses seek for proportionality, taking measures that are essential and effective while working to minimize the negative repercussions of their actions. The ongoing reevaluation of control measures makes it possible to modify ethical standards in accordance with the many conditions that are always changing.

Research Ethics

When doing research with human participants, strict ethical standards are adhered to. This ensures that informed consent is obtained and that risks are kept to a minimum.

Public Engagement in Decision-Making

Ethical avian influenza management includes means
for public engagement in decision-making processes.
Increasing the ethical foundation of control measures
can be accomplished by providing communities with
the ability to actively engage in decision-making.

Education and Outreach Ethics

Ethical education initiatives give truthful information
regarding the risks of avian influenza and the steps that
can be taken to manage it. The practice of
communication is characterized by the respect for
cultural norms and values, the avoidance of
paternalism, and the guarantee that messages will
resonate with a wide range of audiences.

Governmental and International Collaboration

In order to achieve ethical collaboration, it is necessary
for governments and international bodies to share
responsibilities and resources. The provision of
assistance to affected regions and countries in a sense

of global solidarity is an essential component of ethical collaboration during epidemics.

For the purpose of avian influenza management, a complex ethical framework that takes into consideration the interconnectivity of human and animal well-being is required in order to strike a balance between health and animal welfare. In the face of the problems that are posed by avian influenza outbreaks, ethical decision-making requires the navigation of complicated trade-offs, with a priority placed on justice, transparency, and long-term sustainability.

Political and Social Challenges: Navigating Governance and Cooperation

Managing avian influenza is laden with political and social issues that need sophisticated navigation of governance systems and international cooperation. These challenges are a result of the fact that avian influenza is being managed. Addressing the difficulties of avian influenza requires a number of important factors to be addressed, including promoting collaboration across nations, adopting effective legislation, and striking a balance between the interests of many stakeholders.

Intersecting National and Global Interests

Political issues originate from conflicting national priorities, where aspects such as economic considerations, food security, and public health may be in conflict with one another. In order to successfully navigate these issues, it is necessary to encourage global collaboration that is in accordance with the interests of individual nations as well as the larger international aims.

Policy Formulation and Implementation

In order to develop and implement successful policies, it is necessary to coordinate across government departments, including those dealing with health, agriculture, and foreign relations. Political issues develop when policy decisions vary from scientific recommendations, underscoring the significance of evidence-based governance.

Resource Allocation

The execution of comprehensive avian influenza management plans may be hampered by limited resources, which creates political obstacles in the process of resource allocation. In order to successfully navigate resource limits, it is necessary to ensure equal distribution, rectify discrepancies between urban and rural areas, and provide assistance to groups that are currently vulnerable.

Political Will and Commitment

The fact that political leaders are committed to making the control of avian influenza a priority is very necessary for efficient administration. Fostering a long-term vision that acknowledges the significance of persistent efforts beyond immediate crises is necessary in order to successfully navigate the hurdles that are presented by politics.

Global Governance Mechanisms

There is a potential for international collaboration to be hampered when there are no efficient coordination structures at the global level. In order to effectively address political difficulties, it is necessary to enhance international institutions such as the World Health Organization (WHO), the Food and Agriculture Organization (FAO), and the World Organization for Animal Health (OIE).

Openness and Accountability

When there is a lack of openness in the information sharing relationship between nations, political issues might arise. The establishment of accountability measures helps to guarantee that governments comply to international standards and principles that have been agreed upon.

Diplomatic Relations and Cooperation

Geopolitical Considerations should be taken into account while dealing with diplomatic relations and cooperation. It is possible that geopolitical tensions, which restrict international cooperation, may make political difficulties even more difficult to deal with. In order to successfully navigate these hurdles, diplomatic initiatives to encourage cooperation and emphasize shared health security goals involving both parties are required.

Crisis Management and Decision-Making

Political Decision Timeliness: Delays in political decision-making during times of crisis can make the spread of avian influenza much more detrimental. The establishment of expert advisory panels that can provide timely counsel to policymakers during times of emergency is necessary in order to successfully navigate these obstacles.

Social and Cultural Considerations

Political issues may arise when control measures clash with cultural practices relating to the rearing and consumption of poultry by the population. The incorporation of local perspectives through community engagement and the respect of cultural nuances are both necessary components in order to successfully navigate these issues.

International Aid and Cooperation

Political issues occur when countries are dependent on international aid for avian influenza management. In order to successfully navigate these issues, it is necessary to identify and build sustainable funding structures that reduce dependence and guarantee ongoing assistance.

Economic Implications for the Poultry Industry

When avian influenza control measures have an influence on international trade in poultry products, potentially difficult political situations may occur.

In the context of negotiations and agreements: In order to successfully navigate these obstacles, diplomatic talks and trade agreements that strike a balance between concerns about health and economic interests are required.

Capacity Building

Political issues occur owing to inequalities in the capacities of different nations to manage avian influenza. There are a number of international training programs. In order to successfully navigate these hurdles, international collaboration is required to develop capacity in regions with limited resources through the implementation of training programs.

The Position of Non-Governmental Organizations (NGOs):

There is a possibility that political difficulties will emerge if there is opposition to working together with non-governmental organizations. To successfully navigate these issues, it is necessary to acknowledge

the significant role that non-governmental
organizations (NGOs) play and to cultivate
relationships for the purpose of providing reciprocal
support.

National Security Considerations

The perceptions of avian influenza as a danger to
national security may have an impact on the political
problems that are faced. In order to successfully
navigate these obstacles, it is necessary to design risk
mitigation measures that strike a compromise between
matters of public health and concerns of security.

It is necessary to take a comprehensive and cooperative
approach in order to address the political and social
problems that are associated with the control of avian
influenza. In order to improve their resilience and
efficacy in controlling and minimizing the effects of
avian influenza epidemics, governments can improve
their ability to navigate the intricacies of governance,
develop international cooperation, and accommodate
the different interests of stakeholders.

Future Perspectives.

Research Frontiers: Advancements in Bird Flu Studies

In recent years, the study of avian influenza, sometimes known as bird flu, has witnessed major improvements. These advancements have been spurred by research that spans multiple disciplines, technological innovations, and collaborative efforts taken by researchers from all around the world. These new horizons in bird flu research cover a wide range of themes, ranging from the molecular complexities of the virus to the development of innovative ways for the prevention and control of the disease. Our focus here is on the most important research frontiers that have played a significant role in shaping the landscape of bird flu investigations.

Genomic Characterization and Evolution

Recent developments in genomic technology, such as high-throughput sequencing, have made it possible to characterize avian influenza viruses in a manner that is both speedy and complete.

In the field of evolutionary dynamics, the study of the evolution of avian influenza viruses offers valuable insights on the adaptation of these viruses, the patterns of transmission, and the possible risks of zoonotic spillover.

Interactions Between the Host and the Virus

The primary focus of research has been on elucidating the immunological responses of the host to avian influenza. This has helped shed light on both the protective mechanisms and the components that contribute to the pathogenesis of the virus. Investigating the factors that determine the host range of particular avian influenza viruses helps us gain a better understanding of the reasons why these viruses can infect a wide variety of species, including humans.

Identification of zoonotic strains in the zoonotic potential and risk assessment process:

In order to highlight the significance of surveillance and early detection, the purpose of these studies is to identify strains of avian influenza that have the potential to be transmitted from animals to humans. Comprehensive risk assessments investigate the elements that influence the potential of avian influenza spreading to human populations and the chance of this happening.

Virus-Host Dynamics in Wild Bird Populations

Research conducted in wild bird populations sheds light on the ecological dynamics of avian influenza viruses. This research takes into consideration a variety of elements, including migratory patterns, interactions between species, and environmental reservoirs. Collaborative international surveillance networks contribute to the monitoring of avian influenza in wild bird populations. These networks also provide early warning systems for future outbreaks of the disease.

Structural Biology of Avian Influenza Virus

Recent developments in structural biology, in particular Cryo-Electron Microscopy (Cryo-EM), have made it possible for researchers to examine the three-dimensional structures of avian influenza virus components at resolutions that have never been seen before.

By gaining an understanding of the structures of viral proteins, one can gain insights into possible therapeutic targets, which in turn helps to encourage the development of antiviral medications.

Antiviral Drug Development

Researchers are now investigating novel antiviral chemicals that target different stages of the life cycle of the avian influenza virus in an effort to suppress viral replication.

Surveillance of medication resistance helps foresee potential obstacles in the effectiveness of antiviral treatments. These challenges can be anticipated by drug resistance monitoring.

Vaccination Strategies

The development of universal influenza vaccinations that are capable of giving wide protection against a variety of avian influenza strains is the goal of the advancements that have been made in vaccine design.

The primary objective of research is to improve the effectiveness of vaccines and to stimulate powerful immune responses by optimizing adjuvant technologies.

Immune-Escape Mechanisms

By doing research into the antigenic changes of avian influenza viruses, researchers are able to design vaccines that are capable of providing long-term protection against strains that are constantly developing. In order to develop tactics to combat immunological escape mechanisms, it is necessary to have an understanding of how the virus avoids the immune responses of the host.

Epidemiological Modeling and forecast

The incorporation of machine learning and artificial intelligence into epidemiological modeling results in an increase in the accuracy of the forecast of avian influenza outbreaks. In the field of public health, rapid real-time data analysis helps contribute to treatments that are both more effective and more timely.

Biosecurity Measures and Management Strategies

Research analyzes the effectiveness of biosecurity measures in reducing the spread of avian influenza within poultry farms and from wild birds to domesticated birds.

In the context of integrated management approaches, comprehensive management strategies take into account not just virological aspects but also socio-economic and environmental dimensions.

Population Awareness and Risk Communication

Knowing how the general population thinks about and behaves in relation to avian influenza is essential for the development of efficient risk communication methods. In order to encourage proactive participation in avian influenza prevention initiatives, research is being conducted to investigate different types of community engagement.

Community-Based Participatory Research

Community-based participatory research actively incorporates local communities in avian influenza investigations, acknowledging the distinctive knowledge and views that these groups possess. Increasing the capacity of communities to take preventative measures against avian influenza can be accomplished by empowering communities through participation in research.

Research on Global Governance and Policy

Research is conducted to evaluate the effectiveness of national and international policies within the context of preventing and controlling outbreaks of avian influenza. Recommendations for more effective international cooperation in the management of avian influenza are informed by research, which contributes to discussions about global governance.

One Health Integration

Research horizons place an emphasis on the integration of One Health concepts, which encourages collaboration across disciplines in order to address the complex relationships that exist between human, animal, and environmental health.

The research conducted by One Health is used to develop policy recommendations that recognize the interdependence of health systems and argue for holistic approaches to the management of avian influenza.

The advancements that have been made in the field of bird flu research indicate a dynamic field in which continuing study continually enhances our understanding of the virus and informs tactics for prevention, control, and the resilience of global health. It is important to take a collaborative and all-encompassing strategy in order to protect both human and animal populations, and the interdisciplinary nature of these frontiers reflects the concerted effort that is being made to confront the myriad of problems that are faced by avian influenza.

Emerging Threats: Anticipating and Responding to New Challenges

As the landscape of avian influenza continues to evolve, it is essential to anticipate and respond to emerging risks in order to effectively prevent and manage the disease and to ensure the resilience of global health. This all-encompassing investigation dives into the many of facets that comprise the rising dangers in the management of avian influenza. These facets include virological alterations, ecological dynamics, technological hurdles, and the necessity of international cooperation.

Virological Shifts and Genetic Drift:

Mutation Dynamics: It is vital to conduct continuous monitoring in order to monitor genetic changes in avian influenza viruses. These mutations have the potential to influence the transmissibility, aggressiveness, and antigenic features of the virus.

In order to anticipate virological shifts, it is necessary to have an understanding of how viruses adapt to new hosts, which includes the possible dangers of zoonotic infectious transmission.

In order to accurately predict the potential for zoonotic spillover, it is necessary to identify avian influenza strains that possess genetic markers that are associated with enhanced infectivity in humans. It is essential to increase surveillance in both human and avian populations in order to detect zoonotic occurrences at an earlier stage.

Pandemic Preparedness and Global Cooperation

In order to be ready for the possibility of pandemics, it is necessary to engage in scenario planning, which entails taking into consideration a number of different outbreak scenarios and the possible impact they could have on global health. The importance of international cooperation cannot be overstated, and as a result, collaborative structures that enable the exchange of information, the distribution of resources, and the coordination of response operations are required.

Changes in migration patterns

The migration patterns of birds could be altered as a result of climate change, which would have an impact on the geographic distribution of avian influenza viruses. Enhancing ecological resilience and taking into consideration adaptive methods for both wild birds and farmed birds are both necessary steps in the process of preparing for the effects of climate change.

Antiviral Resistance and Treatment Strategies

The development of alternative treatment strategies for antiviral resistance is guided by the proactive monitoring of resistance patterns. Exploring individualized treatment techniques that are tailored to the specific characteristics of avian influenza viruses is an important part of anticipating new dangers.

Public Health Education and Communication

It is essential to become involved in proactive risk communication in order to educate the general public about new dangers and preventative actions.

Surveillance in Wild Bird Reservoirs

Implementing dynamic surveillance networks in wild bird reservoirs boosts early detection capabilities. Having an understanding of the behaviors of wild birds allows for the prediction of probable hotspots and transmission routes.

Policy Adaptation and Governance

In order to anticipate new risks, it is necessary to have governance structures that are equipped with flexible policy frameworks that are able to adjust to changing circumstances. Thus, increasing the extent to which international collaboration platforms are strengthened guarantees coordinated responses and consistent policy execution.

Biological Risk Assessment and Biosafety

The process of conducting comprehensive biological risk assessments is beneficial in detecting potential dangers and putting in place appropriate biosafety measures. In order to anticipate new risks, it is necessary to continuously expand capacity in order to improve biosafety measures on both the local and global levels.

Behavioral Studies and Social Resilience

Behavioral studies contribute to understanding how the public reacts to emerging dangers and inform communication methods. Behavioral studies also contribute to the development of behavioral resilience. Making it possible for communities to have an active role in emergency preparedness and response operations is an essential component of social resilience construction.

Community Engagement and Early Warning Systems

Involving communities in surveillance operations provides an opportunity to build early warning systems that are efficient. In order to anticipate new dangers, it is necessary to have trust-building initiatives in place. These activities should ensure that communities are proactive in reporting and responding to potential outbreaks.

Economic Implications and Livelihood Protection

In order to protect livelihoods, it is necessary to investigate different options for economic diversification within communities that are susceptible to outbreaks of avian influenza. The implementation of insurance and support programs results in a reduction of the economic repercussions that are experienced by farmers and industries that are impacted.

Capacity Building and Training

Strengthening scientific and healthcare capacity globally is crucial for successfully anticipating and responding to new risks. Cross-disciplinary training programs are designed to improve the abilities of professionals who are involved in the management of avian influenza, hence creating a more holistic approach.

In order to anticipate and respond to future dangers in the management of avian influenza, a dynamic and collaborative approach is required. This approach must incorporate scientific innovation, ethical considerations, and global cooperation. In light of the fact that our knowledge of avian influenza is always expanding, it is of the utmost importance to stay one step ahead of new problems in order to guarantee the

health and well-being of animal and human
populations all over the world.

Glossary

A

Antigenic Variation: The ability of a virus, such as avian influenza, to change its surface proteins, making it challenging for the immune system to recognize and respond effectively.

B

Biosecurity: Measures and protocols implemented to prevent the introduction and spread of infectious agents, such as avian influenza, in a defined area, often applied in the context of poultry farms.

C

Culling: The systematic killing of animals, often birds, to control and contain the spread of a disease, such as avian influenza.

E

Eco-Epidemiology: The study of the interactions between ecological processes and the spread of diseases, providing insights into how environmental factors influence the dynamics of avian influenza.

Emerging Threats: Newly identified challenges or risks in avian influenza management that require attention and adaptation of strategies.

G

Genomic Epidemiology: The study of the distribution and determinants of avian influenza at the genomic level, providing insights into the origin, spread, and evolution of the virus.

H

Host Range: The spectrum of hosts that a virus, like avian influenza, can infect and replicate within.

O

One Health Approach: An interdisciplinary approach that recognizes the interconnectedness of human, animal, and environmental health in understanding and addressing diseases such as avian influenza.

P

Pandemic Preparedness: Preparing and planning for a potential global outbreak of avian influenza or other infectious diseases.

R

Real-Time Sequencing: The rapid determination of the genetic sequence of avian influenza viruses, providing up-to-date information for monitoring and responding to outbreaks.

S

Strains and Variants: Different forms or genetic variations of avian influenza viruses that may have distinct characteristics.

T

Transmission Dynamics: The study of how avian influenza spreads among individuals, populations, and regions.

U

Universal Influenza Vaccines: Vaccines designed to provide broad protection against multiple strains of influenza, including various avian influenza strains.

Z

Zoonotic Transmission: The transmission of avian influenza or other diseases from animals to humans.